AF435944

Contents

8 Best Homemade Face Masks for Oily Skin

Oily skin is the most irritating skin type. It catches dirt and impurities very easily from its surroundings and tends to break out. Additional oil secretion demands extra attention for the skin to be healthy and glowing. Homemade face masks can treat many of the problems caused by oily skin, including acne, spots, blackheads, and greasy lines. Though they will give results gradually, unlike other cosmetic beauty treatments, these natural remedies are chemical-free and gentle on the skin.

Gram flour face mask

Gram Flour, Turmeric, Lemon, and Milk Mask

Ingredients

• Two tablespoons gram flour (besan in hindi)

- Five drops of lemon juice

- Half teaspoon of turmeric powder

- Two to three tablespoons of milk

- Water as needed

Directions

Mix ingredients and apply to face for 20 minutes and wash off. It does deep cleansing and removes dead skin cells, giving a clear appearance.

This mask will act as a natural exfoliating scrub for oily skin.

Multani Mitti/Fuller's Earth Face Mask

Homemade multani mitti face masks are very good up soaking up dirt and oil.

Multani mitti, also known as fuller's earth, is an age old remedy used to treat acne and pimples. It's an effective cleanser that can prevent breakouts. You can get rid of extra shine, greasiness and oil with clay masks as they have oil-reducing properties.

A face mask can be made at home with multani mitti as a basic ingredient.

Directions

• Take two tablespoons of fuller's earth powder and soak it in water for half an hour.

• Add a tablespoon of rose water and few drops of lemon juice. If the mixture is still too thick, then you should add some water to it.

• A tablespoon of milk can be added to avoid over-dryness.

• This face mask will clear up your face, improve blood circulation, and remove excess oil and dead cells from skin.

• Apply this clay mask twice or three times a week.

Lemon and Milk to make face pack

Oil-Free Milk and Lemon Mask

Oily skin does need some moisture, but it needs to be oil-free. Milk combined with few drops of lemon makes a mask that is ideal for people with oily skin.

It acts as a natural cleanser. Lemon reduces the oiliness while milk gives the skin a soft and glowing touch of moisture.

Mixture of Rose Water, Glycerin, and Lemon

Mix equal portions of rose water, glycerin and lemon juice and apply to the face. Leave for 20 minutes and wash off.

You can store this lotion in the freezer for daily skin care routine. Keep it in glass bottle.

Lemon has anti-bacterial properties and will help make your skin dry and tight. Rose water is an antiseptic and an excellent cleanser and toner which will give you clean and fresh skin. Glycerin will hydrate the skin.

This is a perfect face mask to treat acne, acne scars and pimples. You must do a patch test to know if this lotion will suit your skin or not.

What type of skin do you have?

• Oily skin

• Dry skin

• Combination skin

• Normal skin

See results

Fruit Face Masks

Lemon, orange, tomato, grapefruit and papaya all benefit oily skin in many ways. They are rich in vitamin C and have astringent oils that are very beneficial for greasy skin.

Natural astringents in these fruits help to tighten facial pores, reduce oil secretion and make skin clean.

People with combination skin should smear these face masks on the T – zone area only (the forehead, nose, and chin). If you apply them on dry areas of your face, then you might suffer from dry patches.

Tomato

Tomato face masks are very effective at dissolving extra oil while shrinking the size of large-looking pores. A tomato has natural astringent properties which make it perfect for this.

Mash a red tomato and apply on face for 15 minutes. You can apply this homemade face mask three times a week.

It will make your skin healthy, toned, and flawless by reducing the appearance of blemishes and acne scars.

Lemon

Lemon does irritate the skin, but at the same time it is very suitable to prevent oily skin problems. Like tomato and papaya, lemon is also rich in vitamin C. The best part of using lemon on your face is its astringent and bleaching effect.

Lemon can be added to face masks prepared at home to deal with all the troubles of greasy and shiny skin, including acne, pimples, blackheads and whiteheads. Your skin will feel clearer, fresh and clean of all the dirt and impurities after using it.

You can apply fresh lemon juice on your skin to clean and reduce oiliness. If your body is oily like your face, then you should add half a lemon to the bathtub to get rid of excessive oil.

Orange Peel

Orange peel is a well-known remedy to manage overly shiny skin.

Orange peels are first dried in the shade and then powdered to make a face mask. It can be used with water, curd, or milk.

Homemade orange peel masks clean and open clogged pores. Its astringent properties also reduces extra oil from the skin.

Papaya

Though papaya suits all skin types, oily skin is most benefited. A papaya face mask will remove excess sebum from the surface of the skin. It also has enzymes that aid in exfoliation treatment.

Using a regular papaya mask on the face means youthful skin, less wrinkles, no dead skin cells and reduced discoloration.

Mash a piece of papaya in a bowl and apply on the face and neck. You can also add few drops of lemon to it.

10 Home Remedies for Oily Skin

Overview

Oily skin is the result of the overproduction of sebum from sebaceous glands. These glands are located under the skin's surface.

Sebum is an oily substance made of fats. Sebum isn't all bad since it helps protect and moisturize your skin and keep your hair shiny and healthy.

Too much sebum, however, may lead to oily skin, which can lead to clogged pores and acne. Genetics, hormone changes, or even stress may increase sebum production.

Oily skin and acne are challenging to manage. Still, home remedies often reduce symptoms without the use of prescription drugs or expensive skin care regimens. Here are 10 remedies for oily skin you can try at home.

1. Wash your face

It seems obvious, but many people with oily skin don't wash their face daily. If your skin's oily, you should wash your face twice a day — but don't overdo it. Avoid harsh soaps or detergents. Use a gentle soap such as glycerin soap instead.

2. Blotting papers

These thin, small papers won't prevent your sebaceous glands from going into overdrive, but they'll allow you to blot excess oil from your face to help minimize shiny, greasy skin. Blotting papers are inexpensive and available over the counter. Use as needed throughout the day.

3. Honey

Honey is one of nature's most revered skin remedies. Thanks to its antibacterial and antiseptic abilities, it may benefit oily and acne-prone skin.

Honey is also a natural humectant, so it helps keep the skin moist but not oily. This is because humectants draw moisture from the skin without replacing it.

To use honey to treat acne and oily skin, spread a thin layer, preferably raw, onto your face; let it dry for about 10 minutes, and rinse thoroughly with warm water.

4. Cosmetic clay

Cosmetic clays, also called healing clays, are used to help absorb skin oil and treat many skin conditions. French green clay is a popular treatment for oily skin and acne since it's highly absorbent. French green clay comes in powder form.

To make a spa-worthy French green clay mask:

1. Add filtered water or rose water to about a teaspoon of clay until it forms a pudding-like consistency.

2. Apply the clay mixture to your face and leave it on until it dries.

3. Remove the clay with warm water and pat dry.

Clay masks removed with water are much gentler on your skin than peel-off masks.

5. Oatmeal

Oatmeal helps calm inflamed skin and absorb excess oil. It also helps exfoliate dead skin. When used in facial masks, oatmeal is usually ground. It can be combined with yogurt, honey, or mashed fruit such as bananas, apples, or papaya. To use oatmeal on your face:

1. Combine 1/2 cup ground oats with hot water to form a paste.

2. Stir in 1 tablespoon honey.

3. Massage the oatmeal mixture into your face for about three minutes; rinse with warm water, and pat dry.

4. Alternatively, apply the oatmeal mixture to your face and leave it on for 10–15 minutes; rinse with warm water, and pat dry.

6. Egg whites and lemons

Egg whites and lemons are a folk remedy for oily skin. Both ingredients are thought to tighten pores. The acid in lemons and other citrus fruits may help absorb oil.

According to a 2008 study, lemons also have antibacterial abilities. However, this remedy is not a good choice for people with egg allergies.

To make an egg white and lemon face mask:

1. Combine 1 egg white with 1 teaspoon freshly-squeezed lemon juice.

2. Apply it to your face, and leave it on until the mask dries.

3. Remove with warm water, and pat dry.

7. Almonds

Ground almonds not only work to exfoliate your skin, but they also help sop up excess oils and impurities. To use an almond face scrub:

1. Finely grind raw almonds to make 3 teaspoons.

2. Add 2 tablespoons of raw honey.

3. Apply to your face gently, in circular motions.

4. Rinse with warm water, and pat dry.

You can also make an almond face mask by grinding the almonds into a paste before adding the honey. Leave the mask on for 10–15 minutes. Rinse with warm water, and pat dry. Do not use if you have a nut allergy.

8. Aloe vera

Aloe vera is known for soothing burns and other skin conditions. According to the Mayo Clinic, there's good scientific evidence that it helps treat flaky skin caused by oily patches. Many people use aloe vera to treat oily skin.

You can apply a thin layer to your face before bedtime and leave it on until morning. Aloe vera is known to cause allergic reaction on sensitive skin. If you have not used aloe vera before, test a small amount on your forearm. If no reaction appears within 24 to 48 hours, it should be safe to use.

9. Tomatoes

Tomatoes contain salicylic acid, a common acne home remedy. The acids in tomatoes may help absorb excess skin oils and unclog pores. To make an exfoliating tomato mask:

1. Combine 1 teaspoon sugar with the pulp of 1 tomato.

2. Apply to the skin in a circular motion.

3. Leave the mask on for 5 minutes.

4. Rinse thoroughly with warm water, and pat dry.

You can also apply just tomato pulp or tomato slices to your skin.

10. Jojoba oil

Although the idea of applying oil to oily skin seems counterproductive, jojoba oil is a folk remedy to treat oily skin, acne, and other skin problems.

It's thought that jojoba mimics sebum on the skin to "trick" sebaceous glands into producing less sebum and help keep oil levels balanced. There's no scientific research to support this theory, though.

Still, a 2012 study found that applying a mask made of healing clay and jojoba oil two to three times weekly helped heal skin lesions and mild acne.

A little jojoba oil goes a long way. Using too much may worsen oily skin. Try massaging a few drops into clean skin a few days a week to see how you react. If you like the results, apply daily.

Preventing oily skin

When oily skin is caused by genetics or hormones, it's tough to prevent. Practicing consistent skin care and avoiding unhealthy foods such as fried foods, foods high in sugar, and processed foods may help.

It's tempting to use heavy cosmetics to cover the effects of oily skin, but this can make the condition worse. When oily skin acts up, reduce the use of makeup, especially foundation. Choose water-based products instead of oil-based. Look for products labeled noncomedogenic that are less likely to clog pores.

Many people claim home remedies for oily skin work. Most remedies aren't well-researched. The success of a home remedy is dependent on many things such as your specific situation and the quality of the products you use.

It's possible to develop allergies to remedies you have been using for a while. If your skin becomes sensitive to any product, discontinue use.

If a home remedy worsens symptoms, stop using it, and contact your doctor or a dermatologist. You should also seek medical help if oily skin symptoms such as acne are severe, since they may lead to infection or scarring.

How To Get Rid Of Oily Skin: 10 Effective DIY Facial Mask Ideas

Having oily skin can be really frustrating. It's hard to keep it clean, or to keep it feeling like it's clean.

Face masks can be helpful for pulling oil out of the skin and making your face look and feel cleaner, but they can be expensive if you use them regularly. These DIY face mask recipes will save you money and give you peace of mind that you're only putting safe ingredients on your face.

Why Oily Skin Happens?

The medical term for oily skin is seborrhea, and it's caused by excess sebum, or skin oil, making your skin look greasy.

Oily skin is often caused by hormones, which is why it often shows up during puberty.[1] An increase in androgen levels during that time of life boost oil production, and while it sometimes goes away once puberty is over, some people are stuck with oily skin.

Having oily skin is genetic, and it can flare up during your period, when you're stressed out, when it's humid outside or when you've done things to produce more oil such as wearing heavy makeup regularly or spending too much time on a dirty cell phone.

If you're too hard on your skin by using harsh cleaning tools, makeup or cleansers that aren't for your skin type or using tanning beds (which dry out the skin, causing it to produce more oil) you can also see oily outbreaks even if you're not genetically predisposed to oily skin. Even some medications can cause your skin to be more oily than normal.

Some of the things that are causing your oily skin might be within your control to change, but if you're still having problems you can try a DIY face mask to help clear up the oil. These recipes use minimal, natural ingredients that won't harm your skin or cause further problems.

Apple Cider Vinegar

A natural antibacterial and antiseptic substance, apple cider vinegar is a great choice for your skin, especially if you have acne as well as oily skin.

Apple cider vinegar can be used alone on your skin; just put some on a cotton ball, apply to your face, let dry and rinse.

You can also use it as a toner, or mix it with baking soda, which has exfoliating properties, to make a mask.

Home Remedies for Life has that recipe as well as other DIY face mask ideas using apple cider vinegar and other ingredients such as sea salt, olive oil and aloe, to name a few.

Banana Face Masks

Another soothing ingredient you can get right at the grocery store that will help your oily skin is banana.

You can simply mash banana and use it alone as a mask, or try one of the recipes from About Beauty. The recipe using banana and honey is the best for oily skin, but any of these would be great for giving your skin a boost.

Really ripe bananas are best for this, and you can even freeze them for a cooling effect on your skin if you want.

Egg White Face Mask

Using egg white on your skin is a great idea because the protein in eggs helps with tissue repair for skin that has been damaged by acne. It's also hydrating and moisturizing and can help slow down the aging process of the skin.

A super simple DIY face mask with egg white is this one from Bellatory that also uses honey and lemon. Honey is antibacterial and lemon juice is an astringent that helps clear out the bacteria that causes acne as well as lightening the skin and evening skin tone.

Oatmeal Face Mask

Add oatmeal to your combination of egg white and honey for an additional exfoliating boost that is great for cleaning and clearing the skin.

Clay and Witch Hazel

Using clay in a DIY face mask is a classic. You won't find this special clay at your regular grocery store, but you can probably find it at a natural foods store or order it online from an herb supplier (or your favorite mega retailer).

The reason bentonite clay is so great for your face is that it draws out impurities. Combine it with witch hazel, as in this recipe from Hello Glow, and you'll have a great astringent, too, which is wonderful for getting the skin clean.

Orange Peel Powder Masks

Another ingredient that is great for the skin but a little harder to come by is orange peel powder. You may be able to find it in the spice section of your grocery store, but it will be less expensive if you buy it from an herbal supplier. You can even make your own orange peel powder by drying and grinding orange peels; check out the how-to from Bellatory.

Whether you buy it or make it yourself, orange peel powder is a great cleanser, astringent and toner that improves circulation and is full of vitamins that encourage healthy skin tone.

The SmartCooky site has a variety of DIY face mask recipes using orange peel powder. The one that includes multani mitti, or fuller's earth, is perfect for oily skin. Multani mitti is a particular kind of clay that has been used in India for generations and is great for removing oil, clearing up acne, evening the skin tone and improving circulation, among other benefits.

Rose Water Face Mask

Another ingredient found in many face mask recipes is rose water. Rose water is actually made from roses, and you can buy it or make your own — this simple tutorial from the Healthy Maven shows you how. It is cleansing, toning and soothing to skin all over the body and is a great addition to bath water as well as to face masks.

Cornmeal and Yogurt Facial Scrub

A quick five-minute mask for oily skin that can be found at Homemade Masks uses yogurt, lemon juice and cornmeal.

Cornmeal is great for exfoliating, while lemon is antiseptic and yogurt helps balance and nourish skin.

Tomato Face Mask Recipes

A surprise ingredient that's actually great to use in homemade face masks is tomatoes. They're as healthy for your skin as they are for the rest of your body.

The vitamins in tomatoes can help fade blemishes and smooth out rough skin, build up collagen to maintain the skin's elasticity and help moisturize your skin, among other things.

Combine tomato with lemon, honey or cucumber depending on your skin's needs with these recipes from Bellatory.

Turmeric Face Mask

Turmeric is the ingredient you want to use for clearing up acne and other skin irritations. It's also great for smoothing out pigmentation irregularities and treating sunburn. And you probably already have some in your spice cabinet!

To make a turmeric face mask like the one at Healthy and Natural World, all you need is turmeric, honey and yogurt. It's a mask that's good enough to eat but you'll want to use it on your face for lots of great benefits.

9 DIY Homemade Face Mask Recipes You Need to Try Tonight

Is your skin acting up? Have you rewatched all seven episodes of Tiger King? Are you pacing around your apartment with no end in sight? Cool, same—that's why we're making DIY face masks tonight. DW, though, I'm not talking about those ~questionable~ recipes you've seen people experimenting with on your Insta feed (lookin' at you, baking soda and lemon juice).

Nope, I went ahead and found nine easy homemade face masks that address everything from rosacea flare-ups to stress-induced breakouts. Keep reading to find the best DIY tutorials for oily skin, acne, blackheads, and more—

all of which you can make with ingredients you def already have in your kitchen. Thankfully.

1. DIY Face Mask for Eczema

This content is imported from YouTube. You may be able to find the same content in another format, or you may be able to find more information, at their web site.

THE INGREDIENTS:

- 1 tablespoon oatmeal

- 1 teaspoon raw honey

- 1/2 teaspoon water

The hero ingredient in this simple DIY is oatmeal, which has both antioxidant and anti-inflammatory properties that help calm dry skin and remove dead skin cells. And when it's coupled with antibacterial honey (and a little h2o for consistency), it's a true skin-soothing treat. Crush up all the ingredients in a bowl, smooth a thin layer over clean skin, and leave it on for about 10 minutes to get the full calming effects.

2. DIY Face Mask for Chapped Lips

Okay, fine, this isn't technically a face mask, but your dry-AF lips need some love, too. Just keep in mind that this recipe from vlogger AnitaSamantha is a bit too abrasive for sensitive or irritated skin, and it should only be used on dry lips once a week. Got it? Cool, go ahead and grab your ingredients:

THE INGREDIENTS:

• 1/2 tablespoon organic cane sugar

• 1/2 tablespoon filtered honey

Yup, all you need is two ingredients for this bb: organic cane sugar (which gives this mask its gritty, exfoliating texture) and filtered honey (which is loaded with antioxidants and helps your skin retain moisture). Mix it up, gently rub the formula along your lips, and rinse it off after five minutes max. Don't forget to follow up with lip balm.

---

3. DIY Face Mask for Dull, Dry Skin

You know those days when your skin just looks...off? Yeah, that's when you need this DIY face mask. It's cooling, calming, and leaves your skin nice and dewy. Don't take it from me, though, because YouTuber

Georgia Peach's perfect skin is pretty much all the evidence you need.

THE INGREDIENTS:

- 1 tablespoon Greek yogurt

- 1 teaspoon oatmeal

- 1 teaspoon honey

Not only does Greek yogurt feel really effing good when you slather it all over your face (just me?), but it's also loaded with things like lactic acid (which helps soften your skin) and probiotics (which helps soothe inflammation). Mix it in a bowl with oatmeal and honey, leave it on clean skin for 10 to 15 minutes, and rinse it off with warm water. Trust: Your skin will feel so damn soft.

4. DIY Face Mask for Acne

Vlogger Nicoletta Xo breaks down four different DIY face masks for acne-prone skin, including a soothing, dark-spot-busting formula that uses nutmeg, honey, and milk, along with a brightening, anti-inflammatory mask with turmeric, yogurt, and honey. But my favorite? This tea tree oil spot-treatment mask.

THE INGREDIENTS:

• 1 tablespoon aloe vera gel

• a drop of tea tree oil

Okay, so on its own, tea tree oil—which is a natural antibacterial and acne-fighter—is way too harsh to slather over your skin (even as a spot treatment, it can quite literally burn your skin if it isn't diluted with enough water). But this mask uses hydrating, calming aloe to negate the potentially irritating effects while calming irritated, broken-out skin. Keep it on clean, dry skin for 10 minutes, then rinse it off, making sure to moisturize afterward.

---

5. DIY Face Mask for Blackheads

In this tutorial, vlogger Ava Jules shows us her favorite DIY face masks, scrubs, and peels, using everything from egg whites (a natural astringent) to my favorite, charcoal powder (an oil absorber), in this DIY mask, below.

THE INGREDIENTS:

• 2 teaspoons unflavored gelatin

• 2 tablespoons water

• 6 activated charcoal capsules (broken open)

Mix all the ingredients together, then dab a relatively thick layer over your nose, basically making your own DIY pore strip (don't worry—this one's significantly more gentle. As a PSA, pore strips can hardcore irritate your skin barrier and actually cause more breakouts and blackheads over time, so skip them and try this instead).

Charcoal works as a natural "magnet" to help draw out and absorb excess oil from your skin, making it excellent for naturally oil, blackhead-prone areas. Just be warned: This mask does dry down into a peel-off mask, so use it only on your nose, where your skin is a bit less sensitive.

---

6. DIY Face Mask for Inflammation

Vlogger SweetPotatoSoul (um, cute) has legit excellent skin, so I'll pretty much try whatever she's suggesting. In this tutorial, she breaks down three different anti-inflammatory masks, my favorite of which uses aloe vera and matcha powder.

THE INGREDIENTS:

• 2 tablespoons fresh aloe (or, in a pinch, aloe vera gel)

• 1 teaspoon matcha green tea powder

Aloe vera is naturally soothing and lightly moisturizing (it's honestly killer for itching and inflamed skin—what up, my rosacea brethren), while matcha powder is believed to have redness-reducing and anti-inflammatory properties. Blend 'em up, slather the mixture on your face (you can stick the mix in the freezer first for 10 minutes for extra cooling powers), leave on for 15 minutes, then rinse off and moisturize.

---

7. DIY Face Mask for Dry Skin

If you have dry skin, you know that the majority of dry-skin remedies involve heavy oils that can also be hella pore-clogging if you're acne-prone. Which is why I'm all for this avocado-and-honey DIY face mask from vlogger Iamvenessae. It's legit only two ingredients and supereasy to recreate at home.

THE INGREDIENTS:

• Half an avocado, mashed

• 1 tablespoon honey

Avocados are full of fatty acids, which help soothe and moisturize your dry skin barrier, while honey is a natural hydrator and astringent (it's been used to treat acne and inflammatory skin conditions without drying out or irritating your skin). Mix and mash the two together, slather all over your face, then wash off after 10 minutes (or 15! Or 20! What a magical life).

---

8. DIY Face Mask for Dark Spots and Acne Scars

Okay, so technically this isn't your classic tutorial video, but it's still really convincing for anyone who deals with hyperpigmentation and acne scars. Vlogger Supa Natural experimented with applying a straight turmeric mask to her skin every day for three days. And, in her words, after three days, "I can see my skin is really calm—the redness is almost gone, and it just feels so smooth, and I'm just happy I did this."

The magical ingredient here is turmeric, which is an antioxidant and anti-inflammatory that's been studied to gently brighten discoloration while killing microorganisms on your skin. Cool, right?

THE (ALTERED) INGREDIENTS:

• 1 teaspoon turmeric powder

• 2 tablespoons plain yogurt (or olive oil, or your favorite face oil)

Although she uses just turmeric and water in the video, I know from experience that applying straight turmeric without a "buffer" can temporarily stain your skin bright yellow. So add a bit of yogurt or oil to create a barrier and prevent any jaundice-lookin' vibes, keep the mixture on your skin for 10 to 15 minutes, then rinse off, followed by your usual face wash.

---

9. DIY Face Mask for Oily Skin

The thing about DIY face masks for oily skin? Then tend to be filled with ultrastripping, ultraharsh ingredients that end up doing more damage than good. But this gentle tutorial from Khichi Beauty uses just two ingredients—egg whites and aloe—to help absorb excess oil without destroying your skin.

THE INGREDIENTS:

• 1 egg white

• 2 tablespoons fresh aloe (or, in a pinch, aloe vera gel)

I know—it sounds super sketch to put raw eggs on your face, but egg whites actually contain a natural antibacterial than can help prevent clogged pores while absorbing excess oil. (No, they won't be as effective as clinically tested and formulated acne treatments, but they also can't hurt, unless you're allergic to eggs.)

And aloe, of course, is an MVP in the calming, soothing, and hydrating departments. So if your skin is overproducing oil as a result of irritation, this two-in-one face mask can help calm it down. Mix the ingredients, spoon them onto your face, hang out for 10 minutes, then rinse them off.

www.ingramcontent.com/pod-product-compliance
Lightning Source LLC
Chambersburg PA
CBHW020939160726
47993CB00007B/2853